The Liberal Case *Against* Abortion

by

Vasu Murti

1ˢᵗ edition published by R.A.G.E. Media, January 2006

Photo Credits:
Unborn Baby Photos (Including Front and Back Cover): Copyright © 2001 Life Issues Institute.
Used with Permission.
"Susan B. Anthony Dollar: Front" (pg 23) © 2004 Jennifer Morgan. Used with Permission.
"Anti-War Protest March" (pg 37) © 2004 Ben Thomas.
Used with Permission.
"Abortion" (pg 48) © 2005 Natalja Sidorenko.
Used with Permission.

ISBN 0-9772234-3-4

To John Morrow,
for opening my eyes to the tragedy of abortion.

Table of Contents

Foreword

In his Farewell Address in 1796, George Washington stated the following about the role religion plays in shaping fundamental moral issues:

"Reason and experience both forbid us to expect that national morality can prevail in exclusion of religious principles."

While this opinion, held by the majority of Washington's contemporaries, has eroded significantly, it is a view commonly held by practitioners of most of the major religions today.

Religion and the belief in an afterlife may make the strongest case to compel believers to *act* upon undoing a wrong, but religion is only one of several persuasions that can make the case for *why* a certain behavior is wrong.

Our awareness about religions of the world has increased proportionately to our increased awareness about cultural diversity. Since Washington's time, advances in technology and communication and the mobility of populations have expanded not only our knowledge of other faiths, but also a greater appreciation for the rights of others to hold differing religious beliefs. Hence, believers in Christianity are challenged by believers in the Jewish tradition. Believers in the Hindu faith are challenged by believers in the tenants of Buddhism. If the challenge is not in the doctrines themselves, the mere presence of their diversity among us demands a more complex response to social problems.

This global awareness of the different perspectives of who God is and what God demands from God's followers, creates a dilemma for governments. Because they are composed of greater and more diverse belief systems, the morality or immorality of certain behaviors is less universally defined. The body politic increasingly experiences tension about how to judge behaviors. Without a common determination of how actions effect for ill or well the greater good, modifications in conduct may be less likely to occur, or may even not occur at all.

If there is one universal law that is common to most religions it is the ethic of reciprocity, that one treats others as one wants to be treated:

Hinduism: "Do naught unto others which would cause you pain if done unto you."

Judaism: "What is hateful to you, do not to your fellow man. This is the law."

Christianity: "In everything, do unto others as you would like them to do unto you."

Humanism: "Don't do things you wouldn't want to have done to you."

Cultures whose various religions demand that they love their neighbor as themselves are irreconcilably challenged by ever evolving and devolving bodies of religious thought. How does one interpret who is one's neighbor? How does one's self choose to be treated? How does one extend that concern to others? How far is one compelled to extend that concern?

The diversity of answers to these questions posed by the myriad of concepts of who God is demands a new paradigm. Too much is at stake to not strive to meet this challenge.

The crisis of who will live and who will die underpins this challenge. Wars rage, and often do so even in the name of religion. Civil and global strife directly deprive millions of their very lives. Killing in the name of personal or national security occurs through capital punishment, abortion, and endless incidences of torture and environmental destruction. Indirect killing occurs through the '*isms*' that diminish human rights or the quality of life of civil society: capitalism, sexism, ageism, racism, and classism.

Add to this the emergence of a body of thought that does not believe in a higher power that directs our behavior, or to whom we are responsible. Are atheists exempted from universal truths? Or can atheists lend an understanding to the development of these truths and the observance of right and wrong?

Religion should never cease to amplify answers about how to treat others as one wants to be treated. But this universal question can no longer be left in its entirety to religion alone.

Murti attempts to explore, without religion, one of the most contentious issues of our day: the question of abortion. For as much as the atomic bomb forever altered questions about war and peace, so has abortion forever altered the meaning of human life and our responsibility to it. By creatively and passionately using the universal question of the rights of animals, Murti analyzes the rights of the unborn. The power of his persuasion is not based on one or more bodies of religious thought, but on sentient beings' natural tendency to protect one another.

3

For too long has the discussion of these questions been relegated to religious beliefs. For too long has there been only feeble attempts to find a greater common denominator to solicit understanding between their relationship. For too long has there been bodies of fragmented thought that pit the rights of one over and above the rights of the other.

It may be assuming too much to expect that the readers of this work will value both the life of other animals and the life of an unborn human being equally. Perhaps like myself, you too are on a journey seeking to approach the radical center point where their equality meet.

The contribution of this book is that it removes divisive faith beliefs surrounding their inequality, and searches for and presents grounded reasoning for their equality using universal argumentation common to any person of faith or to a person of no faith.

Religious principles must not be abandoned, or replaced, or deleted. Rather we recognize here that argumentation can be enhance with secular and scientific principles. This strategy can serve as a guideline to many religious institutions today. For instance, many bodies of faith are quick to point out that they believe abortion is morally wrong in the majority of cases. Other religions may maintain that killing animals for food, clothing, or sport is morally wrong. However, these voices have been silenced by critics who claim it is inappropriate for the religious view of moral conduct to be shared in the marketplace of ideas. This is self-censorship that attempts to make religion irrelevant.

However, if universal arguments can serve to enhance a religious position, that position will become more universally accepted. For instance, the onset of human life is not a dogma of religion but a fact of science. The humanity of the unborn does not have to be found in the Bible or the Koran. It can be found in a college textbook on embryology.

How much more convenient for the perils of the ethic of reciprocity if we needed to rely on religion instead of human genetic engineering. In Galileo's era, religion was criticized for not recognizing scientific information. Today, can religion be criticized when it insists on, when it demands, that society recognize science?

Once terms of common understanding about life are established, the moral *why* will be answered. That will then allow the convictions of religious and humanist alike to act upon a course of moral conduct to protect both the rights of animals and of unborn human beings.

Carol Crossed

President, Democrats for Life of America

Alive and Kicking

Abortion policy must be completely secular. In 1797, America made a treaty with Tripoli, declaring that "the government of the United States is not, in any sense, founded on the Christian religion." This reassurance to Islam was written under Washington's presidency and approved by the Senate under John Adams.

Dr. Bernard Nathanson, a physician who presided over 60,000 abortions before changing sides on the abortion issue, wrote in his 1979 book *Aborting America*: "The U.S. statutes against abortion have a non-sectarian history. They were put on the books when Catholics were a politically insignificant minority... even the Protestant clergy was not a major factor in these laws. Rather, the laws were an achievement of the American Medical Association.

"Traditionally, religion opposes abortion because 'the Lord giveth, the Lord taketh away.' What about atheists like myself who do not believe in the existence of a personal God? I think that abortion policy ought not be beholden to a sectarian creed... In the case of abortion, however, we can and must decide on the biological evidence... without resorting to scriptures, revelations, creeds, hierarchical decrees, or belief in God. Even if God does not exist, the fetus does."

In 1827, Von Baer determined fertilization to be the starting point of individual human life. By the 1850s, medical communities were advocating legislation to protect the human unborn. In 1859, the American Medical Association protested legislation which protected the human unborn only after "quickening."

A rational, secular case thus exists for the rights of the human unborn. Individual human life is a continuum from fertilization until death. Zygote, embryo, fetus, infant, toddler, adolescent, adult, etc. are all different stages of human development. To destroy that life at any stage of development is to destroy that individual. The real question in the abortion debate is not the seemingly absurd scenario of giving full human rights to human zygotes, but rather the thorny question of how to legally protect those rights without violating a new mother's privacy and civil liberties. And the right to privacy is not absolute. If parents are abusing an already born child, for example, government "intrusion" is warranted – children have rights.

Recognizing the rights of another class of beings limits our freedoms and our choices and requires a change in our lifestyle – the abolition of (human) slavery is a good example of this. A 1964 New Jersey court ruling required a pregnant woman to undergo blood transfusions – even if her religion forbade it – for the sake of her unborn child. One could argue, therefore – apart from religion – that recognizing the rights of the human unborn, like the rights of blacks, women, lesbians and gays, children, animals, and the environment, is a sign of secular social progress.

The humanity of the unborn: Are the unborn human? Yes. Biologically, the unborn are not only human, they have an individual human genetic identity; 46 human chromosomes. Virtually all medical authorities (physicians, biologists, etc.) agree with geneticist Ashley Montagu who wrote: "The fact is simple. Life begins not at birth, but at conception." J. Lejeune of Paris, discoverer of the chromosome pattern of Down's syndrome, observed: "Each individual has a very neat beginning, at conception."

When does human life begin? "At conception," states Professor W. Bowes of the University of Colorado. Professor M. Matthews-Roth of Harvard writes: "It is scientifically correct to say that individual human life begins at conception." Dr. Mary Calderon of Planned Parenthood in the 1960s, wrote: "Fertilization has taken place; a baby has been conceived."

Everything that defines a person physically is present at fertilization – only oxygen, nutrients and time to develop are required. The unborn child has his or her own genetic code, EEG trackings, and circulatory system. Often, the blood type and sex of the unborn child will also differ from that of the mother. The heart of the unborn child begins beating at 18 days, and is pumping blood at 21 days. The brain is functioning at 40 days – EEG trackings have been made at less than six weeks gestation. The unborn child responds to stimuli by the sixth to eighth week. Rapid Eye Movements (REMs) characteristic of actual dream states, are present in 23 weeks. There are clearly *two* distinct individuals (mother and child) present during pregnancy.

Philosophical debates about the "personhood" of the human unborn resemble the old, medieval arguments about ensoulment. Dr. J.C. Willke, former head of National Right to Life, summarizes the case against abortion as follows:

"Ask the question, is this fertilized ovum alive? Yes, by any dimension of that word, this fertilized ovum is alive, growing, replacing multiplying cells, life. Is this fertilized ovum human? How can you tell a human from a rabbit, from a carrot? Genetic chromosomes. Take a look, 46 human chromosomes, this is a member of the human species. This is human, growing, intact, programmed from within, moving forward in a self-controlled ongoing process of maturation, development, sexed male or female, replacement of his or her own dying cells, within ten days taking control of the host body that this little being grows within, controlling physiologically the host body for the balance of that gestation time, enlarging her breasts, softening her pelvic bones, setting his own birthday, all this controlled by the developing baby, this is alive, human and sexed.

"That's the biological measurement. Total intactness from a single cell. You're 40 million million cells, but every single cell is the identical replication, genetically speaking, of the first one. Nothing was added to that single cell, who you once were, nothing but nutrition. Biologically, there isn't a perception, there isn't an opinion, biological, it's absolute...

"What are the other yardsticks? They all fall into a category that can be described as philosophic theories. This is not human until an exchange of love, until a certain degree of consciousness, until a certain degree of maturation, until a certain degree of independence, viability, until birth... certain IQ, whatever. Now, all of those are used as yardsticks to define the word 'human life' or if you please, 'person.' Now the question is, what do they all have in common? Not one is subject to natural science and proof. They are all beliefs or theories. People of good will differ diametrically upon these and if you put six such people in the room, you might get six different answers.

"We believe the yardsticks of philosophic measurement of the word 'human life' should be subject to the same political judgment as the religious beliefs on human life and just as we should not impose a religious faith, belief upon our neighbors through force of law, so we should not impose a philosophic theory upon our neighbors through force of law... we would go back to the one area that we cannot disagree on, that is the biologic judgment, and we would say that the... question, is this human life, should be answered scientifically."

"I will maintain the utmost respect for human life, from the time of conception; even under threat, I will not use my medical knowledge contrary to the laws of humanity."

---Declaration of Geneva
   World Medical Association
   September, 1948

"The child, by reason of his physical and mental immaturity, needs special safeguards and care, including appropriate legal protection, before as well as after birth."

---A Declaration of the Rights of the Child
   United Nations General Assembly
   1959

"Is birth control an abortion?"

"Definitely not. An abortion kills the life of a baby after it has begun."

---Planned Parenthood pamphlet
   August 1963

"Every person has the right to have his life respected, this right shall be protected by law and, in general, from the moment of conception. No one shall be arbitrarily deprived of his life."

---American Convention on Human Rights in San Jose
   November 22, 1969

"The reverence of each and every human life has been the keystone of Western medicine... it has been necessary to separate the idea of abortion from the idea of killing, which continues to be socially abhorrent. The result has been a curious avoidance of the scientific fact, which everyone really knows, that human life begins at conception and is continuous, whether intra- or extra-uterine. The very considerable semantic gymnastics which are required to rationalize abortion as anything but taking a human life would be ludicrous if they were not put forth under socially impeccable auspices."

---Editorial,
Journal of the California State Medical Association
September 1970

In one anti-abortion pamphlet, Dr. Jean Garton states that religion did not discover when human life begins, the biologists did. The fact that religious people may oppose abortion does not make abortion a "religious" issue any more than the fact that religious people may oppose drunk driving makes drunk driving a "religious" issue. In her book, *Who Broke the Baby?*, Dr. Garton compares discrimination against the human unborn to other forms of discrimination:

"By placing unborn human beings *outside* the protection of the law, it became possible to deny them basic rights. This is not the first time in our history that we have made a distinction between the biological category of living human beings and the legal concept of 'person.' At one time in our history American Indians were not legal persons because we did not grant them the protection of our

Constitution. Thus we were able to take by force anything which belonged to them.

"Usually what we wanted was their land, so we denied them the right to property. Next in our national list of non-persons were black slaves, declared to be chattel and property of their masters as a result of the *Dred Scott* decision of 1857... In 1973, another group of human beings was added to the non-person list: the unborn."

Prenatal Development

Information adapted from the Medical Encyclopedia *of the U.S. National Library of Medicine. Photos courtesy of Life Issues Institute's* "Windows to the Womb" *prenatal photo collection.*

Day One: The sperm and the ovum, each containing 23 chromosomes, unite to form a single embryo with 46 chromosomes – the number of chromosomes that identifies an organism as human. The unique DNA for the individual is also formed, containing the genetic code that will uniquely identify the person for their entire life.

Week 3: The heart, brain, spinal cord and digestive tract begin to develop.

Weeks 4 to 5: The heart begins to beat; fluid begins to flow through the blood vessels.

Week 6: Feet and hands are distinguishable. Brain activity can be measured.

Week 7: All organs have begun to form; hair follicles form.

Photo Taken at Seven Weeks

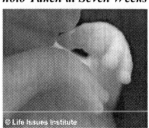

© Life Issues Institute

Weeks 9 to 12 (end of first trimester): The face is now well-formed, tooth buds appear. The child can now make a fist. Red blood cells are being produced, and the sex of the child can now be determined via ultrasound.

Weeks 13 to 16: Sucking motions are made with the mouth, as well as other active movement now that muscle tissue has formed and bones have developed. The liver and pancreas are now functioning.

Week 20: Fingernails, eyebrows and eyelashes appear. The mother can usually feel the baby moving, and the heartbeat can be heard with a stethoscope.

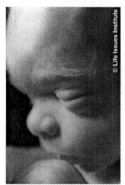

Photo Taken at 20 Weeks

Week 24 (end of second trimester): The eye is developed, and a startle reflex is noticeable. Footprints and fingerprints form.

Weeks 25 to 28: The lungs are now capable of breathing, though not necessary in the mother's womb. The nervous system is developed enough for some voluntary motion, and the eyelids can open and close. Survival outside the mother is now possible, though dangerous.

Week 37 to 40(end of third trimester): The pregnancy is considered full term at 37 weeks.

Additional Photos of Prenatal Development

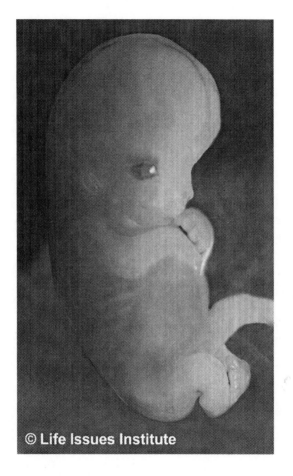

Photo Taken at Seven Weeks

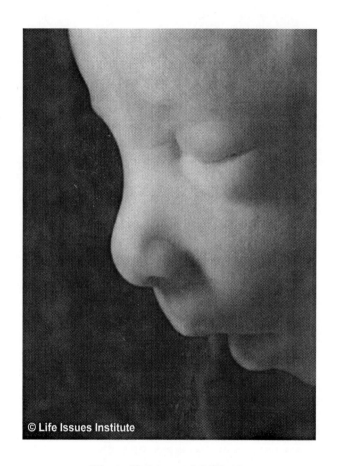

Photo Taken at 16 Weeks

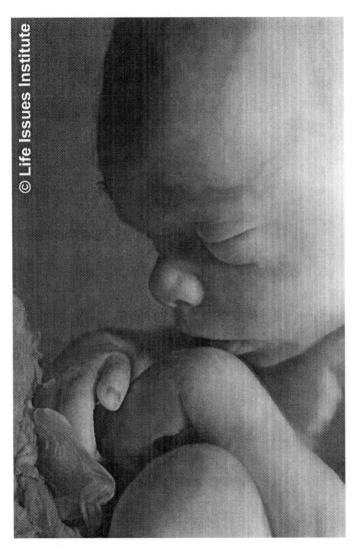

Photo Taken at 20 Weeks

Nonviolent Femmes

According to contemporary pro-life feminist Mary Krane Derr, "The debate raging over abortion today is not the first one in American history; there was one during the Victorian era."

Derr writes that despite the large monetary loss involved, *The Revolution*, the suffragist paper put out by Susan B. Anthony and Elizabeth Cady Stanton refused to run ads for patent medicines because these were frequently thinly disguised abortifacients.

A similar policy was practiced by *Woodhull's and Claflin's Weekly*, the paper published by free love advocates Victoria Woodhull and Tennessee Claflin. The *Weekly* constantly attacked Madame Restell, a well known New York City abortionist. Victoria Woodhull, the first woman to attempt to run for President, was a fierce opponent of abortion. The *Weekly* (December 24, 1870) proclaimed, "The rights of children as individuals begin while yet they remain the foetus."

According to Woodhull: "Men must no longer insult all womanhood by saying that freedom means the degradation of woman. Every woman knows that if she were free, she would never bear an unwished-for child, nor think of murdering one before its birth." (*Evening Standard*, November 17, 1875)

"Victorian feminists," Derr observes, "were highly critical of Victorian sexual ethics. They affirmed the value of sex for pleasure and communication as well as procreation, for men and women alike... they celebrated motherhood itself as a uniquely female power and strength which deserved genuine reverence."

According to Derr, "From early in the 19th century, Americans – even lay people – were exposed to enough information about embryology to enable them to make a critical and ethically significant distinction between contraception and abortion: the former practice did not terminate a human life but the latter one did."

In *The Radical Remedy in Social Science* (1886), feminist and civil libertarian Edward Bond Foote crusaded for public and legal acceptance of contraception, insisting it would not only promote the well-being of women, but that it would also reduce the destruction of unborn children, which he termed "a wastefulness of human life."

Susan B. Anthony called abortion "child-murder" and insisted, "We want *prevention*, not merely punishment. We must reach the root of the evil... It is practiced by those whose inmost souls revolt from the dreadful deed." Anthony recognized that one of the root causes of abortion was the male exploitation of women: "All the articles on this subject that I have read have been from men. They denounce women as alone guilty, and never include man in any plans for the remedy." (*The Revolution*, July 8, 1869)

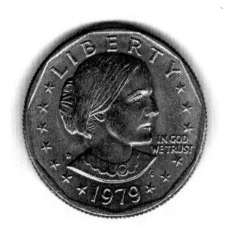

Susan B. Anthony, feminist pioneer, suffragist, and anti-slavery advocate, was the first real woman to be honored by having her portrait placed on U.S. currency. She also referred to abortion as "child-murder."

Like Susan B. Anthony, Matilda Gage also held men accountable: "[This] subject lies deeper down in woman's wrongs than any other... I hesitate not to assert that most of [the responsibility for] this crime lies at the door of the male sex." (*The Revolution*, April 9, 1868)

Elizabeth Cady Stanton classified abortion along with the killing of newborns as "infanticide." (*The Revolution*, February 5, 1868) According to Stanton: "When we consider that women are treated as property, it is degrading to women that we should treat our children as property to be disposed of as we see fit." (Letter to Julia Ward Howe, October 16, 1873)

Stanton not only opposed abortion, but recognized the social factors causing women to seek it: "There must be a remedy even for such a crying evil as this," she wrote. "But where shall it be found, at least where begin, if not in the complete enfranchisement and elevation of women?" (*The Revolution*, March 12, 1868)

Mattie Brinkerhoff also recognized that social factors such as poverty and discrimination cause women to seek abortions:

"When a man steals to satisfy hunger, we may safely conclude that there is something wrong in society – so when a woman destroys the life of her unborn child, it is an evidence that either by education or circumstances she has been greatly wronged... How shall we prevent this destruction of life and health? By the true education and independence of woman." (*The Revolution*, September 2, 1869)

"Child murderers," wrote Sarah Norton, "practice their profession without let or hindrance, and open infant butcheries unquestioned... Is there no remedy for all this ante-natal child murder?... Perhaps there will come a time when... an unmarried mother will not be despised because of her motherhood... and when the right of the unborn to be born will not be denied or interfered with." (*Woodhull and Claflin's Weekly*, November 19, 1870)

Even into the 20th century, feminists continued to oppose abortion as an *injustice* towards women rather than a means to their emancipation.

"The custom of procuring abortions has reached such appalling proportions in America as to be beyond belief..." wrote anarchist Emma Goldman in *Mother Earth* in 1911. "So great is the misery of the working classes that seventeen abortions are committed in every one hundred pregnancies."

Alice Paul, the author of the original Equal Rights Amendment (ERA) in 1923, opposed the later trend of linking it with abortion rights. She insisted that "abortion is the ultimate exploitation of women."

Whether for public relations purposes or her actual heartfelt feelings, Margaret Sanger, founder of the American Birth Control League (now known as Planned Parenthood), expressed opposition to abortion. She lamented the resort of poor people to "the most barbaric method" of family planning, "the killing of babies—

infanticide – abortion." (*My Fight for Birth Control*, 1931) Sanger told clients in her first birth control clinic that "abortion was the wrong way – no matter how early it was performed it was taking a life." (*An Autobiography*, 1938)

Although Simone de Beauvoir supported the legalization of abortion, she described it as an injustice to women: "Men tend to take abortion lightly; they... fail to realize the values involved. The woman who has recourse to abortion is disowning feminine values, her values... Women learn to believe no longer in what men say... the one thing they are sure of is this rifled and bleeding womb, these shreds of crimson life, this child that is not there." (*The Second Sex*, 1952)

A 1972 Presidential commission on population growth recommended legalizing abortion, with only a few voices dissenting. One of those voices expressing opposition to legalized abortion was Graciela Olivarez, a Chicana active in civil rights and anti-poverty work. "The poor cry out for justice and equality," she lamented, "and we respond with legalized abortion. I believe that in a society that permits the life of even one individual (born or unborn) to be dependent on whether that life is 'wanted' or not, all its citizens stand in danger... We do not have equal opportunities. Abortion is a cruel way out."

In 1972, the National Organization for Women (NOW) expelled all its pro-life members in order to stifle dissent on the abortion issue. These pro-life feminists went on to form their own organization. Feminists For Life now has chapters in the United States, Canada and New Zealand.

In her article "Feminism and Abortion: The Great Inconsistency" (*The New Zealand Listener*, January 7, 1978), Daphne de Jong responded to the pro-abortion argument that the unborn child is merely part of its mother and not a separate individual human being endowed with human rights:

"Until this century, the laws of both Britain and America made women a 'part of' their husbands.

"'By marriage, the husband and wife are one person in law... our law in general considers man and wife one person.' (Blackstone's *Commentaries*, 1768)

"The one person was, of course, the husband, who exerted absolute power over his wife and her property. She had no existence and therefore no protection under the law. The only thing a husband could not do was kill her.

"The earliest feminist battles were fought against the legal chattel status of women. Many feminists were among those who overturned the U.S. Supreme Court decision of 1857, that a black slave was 'property' and not entitled to the protection of the Constitution.

"Feminism totally rejected the concept of ownership in regard to human beings. Yet when the Court ruled in 1973 that the fetus was the property of its mother, and not entitled to the protection of the Constitution, 'liberated' women danced in the streets."

In an article entitled "Pro-Abortionists Poison Feminism," which appeared in the *Tallahassee Democrat*, Rosemary Bottcher described abortion as a form of discrimination:

"Pro-abortion feminists resent the discrimination against a whole class of humans because they happen to be female, yet they themselves discriminate against a whole class of humans because they happen to be very young.

"They resent that the value of a woman is determined by whether some man wants her, yet they declare that the value of an unborn child is determined by whether some woman wants him. They resent that women have been 'owned' by their husbands, yet insist that the unborn are 'owned' by their mothers.

"They believe that a man's right to do what he pleases with his own body cannot include the right to sexually exploit women, yet proclaim that a woman's similar right means that she can kill her unborn child."

In an article entitled "Pro-Life, Pro-ERA," appearing in *Pro-Life Feminism: Different Voices* (1985), Juli Loesch wrote about an ardent Feminists For Life caucus "calling for a new amendment combining both the ERA, and the HLA (Human Life Amendment), a sort of Equal Human Life Rights Amendment: to 'ensure equality of rights under the law for all persons, regardless of sex, from fertilization to natural death.'"

Pro-Life Feminism: Different Voices contains observations by numerous pro-life feminists on the subject of abortion. According to these pro-life feminists, abortion is not the answer to the problem of unwanted pregnancy, it is merely a band-aid which prevents real reforms from taking place regarding society's treatment of women.

Susan Maronek, for example, writes: "Abortion, in the final analysis, works to the advantage of the exploitative male, not for the female. It provides an end to any and all financial, legal or social obligation which comes with childbirth by eliminating the possibility of birth. Abortion provides the ultimate rationale when pressing for sexual favors. It makes the female a perpetual and re-usable sex object. When an unwanted pregnancy occurs, the female is potentially left without any social support.

"The male can remove himself from the situation, physically or mentally because abortion is 'her' right. The female is left with the sole and final legal responsibility for killing their offspring. It is her body and mind which bear the scars of this destructive operation and experience... Abortion is a male sexual fantasy come true."

Pregnancy and childbirth are *natural*. The ability to bear children is the one thing which truly distinguishes women from men. Demanding the right to abort in order to achieve equality implies women must become males in order to compete and survive in a man's world. Rosemary Bottcher points out that abortion reduces women to the status of sex machines which can be "repaired," if necessary. She refers to it as the "castration of women."

"What we need now," writes Jo McGowan, "is a race of woman who will stand up and say NO! The violence ends here. The misogyny ends here. The destruction of our children ends here. No longer will our bodies be used to write messages of fear and hatred. We hold within our bodies the power of creation, the power to nourish and sustain life. We shall not pervert these to serve death."

"Abortion is the destruction of human life and energy that does nothing to eradicate the very real underlying problems of women," writes Cecilia Voss Koch. "The pregnant welfare mother begs for decent housing, a decent job and childcare or respect for her child-nurturing work. Instead, she gets direction to the local abortion clinic and is told to take care of 'her problem.' How convenient. Much less time and trouble than teaching her about authentic reproductive freedom and reproductive responsibility. Much cheaper than attending to her real problems: her poverty, her lack of skills, her illiteracy, her loneliness, her bitterness about her entrapment, her self-contempt, her vulnerability. After the abortion, these problems will all be there...

"By encouraging society to consider a woman's child as a disposable piece of property, aborting reinforces the image of woman herself as disposable property and reusable sex object – a renewable resource. It is no coincidence that the biggest single financial contributor to the cause of 'abortion rights' is the Playboy Foundation. When abortion is available to all women, all male responsibility for fertility control has been removed. A man need only offer a woman money for the abortion and that's it: no responsibility, no relationship, no commitment. And there we are – recycled and used again!"

Feminist writer Mary Ann Schaefer refers to pro-abortion feminism as "terrorist feminism" because you have to be "willing to kill for the cause you believe in."

Abortion, of course, merely reflects a larger problem. Abortion is *symptomatic* of the rampant sexism within our society – it is not the cure. Television advertisements, sitcoms, women's books, magazines, etc. are still sexist in nature.

Most imply that women are nothing more than homemakers, or that their only goal in life is to catch a man. Women still earn only 60 cents for every dollar a man makes. The average pay of female college graduates is equivalent to that of males who graduated from high school. Only 0.8 percent of all working women earn over $25,000 per year.

The majority of working women are unorganized and underpaid. Working mothers are also forced to pay for childcare and still tend to be segregated into women's jobs. A 1981 survey, for example, found that 75 percent of all practicing physicians were male. Abortion itself is a huge practice run by entrepreneurs – mostly males – with $320 million in yearly profits. "If women must submit to abortion to preserve their lifestyle or career, their economic or social status," writes Daphne de Jong, "they are pandering to a system devised and run by men for male convenience."

"Collectively, society is eroded by abortion," writes Juli Loesch. "Society at large can say: 'Lady, we feel no particular responsibility for your little problem because there is nothing to feel responsible for; so just terminate your problem and everybody will breathe easier.' Lacking the secure base of a caring community, women whose pregnancies are an emotional, social or financial burden are thrown onto the demands of a rather heartless individualism."

In a 1989 opinion editorial on the subject of abortion entitled "The Bitter Price of Choice," pro-life feminist Frederica Matthewes-Green, wrote: "It is a cruel joke to call this a woman's 'choice.' We may choose to sacrifice our life and career plans, or choose to undergo humiliating invasive surgery and sacrifice our offspring. How fortunate we are – we have a choice! Perhaps it's time to amend the slogan – 'Abortion: a woman's right to capitulate.'"

In her article, "The Feminist Case *Against* Abortion," which originally appeared in the September 13, 1999 issue of *The Commonwealth*, Serrin Foster, Executive Director of Feminists For Life, wrote: "The feminist movement was born more than two hundred years ago when Mary Wollstonecraft wrote *A Vindication of the Rights of Woman*. After decrying the sexual exploitation of women, she condemned those who would 'either destroy the embryo in the womb, or cast it off when born.' Shortly thereafter, abortion became illegal in Great Britain.

"The now revered feminists of the 19th century were also strongly opposed to abortion because of their belief in the worth of all humans. Like many women in developing countries today, they opposed abortion even though they were acutely aware of the damage done to women through constant child-bearing. They opposed abortion despite knowing that half of all children born died before the age of five. They knew that women had virtually no rights within the family or the political sphere. *But they did not believe abortion was the answer.*

"Ironically," noted Foster, "the anti-abortion laws that early feminists worked so hard to enact to protect women and children were the very ones destroyed by the *Roe v.*

Wade decision 100 years later – a decision hailed by the National Organization for Women (NOW) as the 'emancipation of women.'

"The goals of the more recent NOW-led women's movement with respect to abortion would have outraged the early feminists," concluded Foster. "What Elizabeth Cady Stanton called a 'disgusting and degrading crime' has been heralded by Eleanor Smeal, former president of NOW and current president of the Fund for a Feminist Majority, as a 'most fundamental right.'"

Pro-Life Liberals

In an article appearing in the September 1980 issue of *The Progressive* entitled, "Abortion: The Left Has Betrayed the Sanctity of Life," Mary Meehan wrote:

"If much of the leadership of the pro-life movement is right-wing, that is due largely to the default of the Left. We little people who marched against the war and now march against abortion would like to see leaders of the Left speaking out on behalf of the unborn. But we see only a few, such as Dick Gregory, Mark Hatfield, Richard Neuhaus, Mary Rose Oakar. Most of the others either avoid the issue or support abortion.

"We are dismayed by their inconsistency. And we are not impressed by arguments that we should work and vote for them because they are good on such issues as food stamps and medical care...

"It is out of character for the Left to neglect the weak and the helpless. The traditional mark of the Left has been its protection of the underdog, the weak, and the poor. The unborn child is the most helpless form of humanity, even more in need of protection than the poor tenant farmer or the mental patient or the boat people on the high seas. The basic instinct of the Left is to aid those who cannot aid themselves – and that instinct is absolutely sound. It is what keeps the human proposition going."

Meehan stated elsewhere that:

"Writer and activist Jay Sykes, who led Eugene McCarthy's 1968 antiwar campaign in Wisconsin and later served as head of the state's American Civil Liberties Union, wrote a 'Farewell to Liberalism' several years ago. Sykes cited several areas of disagreement and disillusionment, then added, 'It is on the abortion issue that the moral bankruptcy of contemporary liberalism is most clearly exposed.' He said that liberals' arguments in support of abortion 'could, without much refinement, be used to justify the legalization of infanticide.'"

In her article, "Abortion and the Left" which originally appeared in *Religious Socialism* (Spring, 1981), Juli Loesch, founder of Pro-Lifers for Survival (an anti-nuclear group) described the response to Mary Meehan's article in *The Progressive*:

"The Left... is profoundly divided on abortion... in October 1980, Pax Christi USA, a Catholic peace organization that includes feminists and socialists, approved an anti-abortion resolution at its national assembly by virtually unanimous vote.

"Weeks later, *Sojourners*, a Christian peace/justice magazine, featured Daniel Berrigan, Shelley Douglass, Jesse Jackson and others arguing for opposition to abortion integrated with a more radical commitment to non-violent feminism and human dignity.

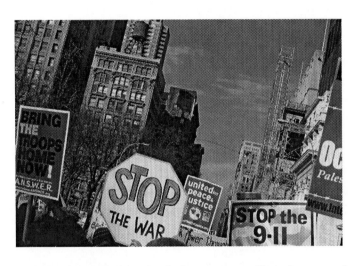

Why is it the Left as a whole protests all violations of human rights, war, and loss of life, championing the underdog and those who cannot speak for themselves – except the unborn?

"Possibly abortion never was a Left/Right issue," concluded Loesch. "Soon after the 1973 *Roe v. Wade* decision one of the most progressive Senate Democrats, Harold Hughes, joined one of the most progressive Republicans, Mark Hatfield, in co-sponsoring a Human Life Amendment (HLA). Both were opponents of the Vietnam War. Both opposed abortion because of, not despite, their other political views... Michael Harrington once called pro-life one of the only true grassroots movements to emerge from the '70s."

"I have always thought it peculiar how the liberal and conservative philosophies have lined up on the abortion issue," observed Rosemary Bottcher in her article "How Do Pro-Choicers 'Fool' Themselves?" which originally appeared in the *Tallahassee Democrat*.

"It seemed to me that liberals traditionally have cared about others and about human rights, while conservatives have cared about themselves and property rights. Therefore, one would expect liberals to be defending the unborn and conservatives to be encouraging their destruction."

Rosemary Bottcher criticized the American Left for its failure to take a stand against abortion:

"The same people who wax hysterical at the thought of executing, after countless appeals, a criminal convicted of some revolting crime would have insisted on his mother's unconditional right to have him killed while he was still innocent.

"The same people who organized a boycott of the Nestle Company for its marketing of infant formula in underdeveloped lands would have approved of the killing of those exploited infants only a few months before.

"The same people who talk incessantly of human rights are willing to deny the most helpless and vulnerable of all human beings the most important right of all.

"Apparently these people do not understand the difference between contraception and abortion," concluded Bottcher. "Their arguments defending abortion would be perfectly reasonable if they were talking about contraception. When they insist upon 'reproductive freedom' and 'motherhood by choice' they forget that 'pregnant' means 'being with child.' A pregnant woman has already reproduced; she is already a mother."

At a speech before the National Right to Life Convention in Cherry Hill, New Jersey, on July 15, 1982, Reverend Richard John Neuhaus of the Evangelical Lutheran Church said:

"I have a confession to make. I am a liberal. More than that. I am a Democrat... I know that among some pro-life advocates liberalism is almost a dirty word. I know it and I regret it. I know that among others there has been a determined effort to portray the pro-life movement as anti-liberal and, indeed, as reactionary. I know it and I regret it.

"We are today engaged in a great contest over the meaning of liberalism, over the meaning of liberal democracy, indeed over the meaning of America... Will it be an America that is inclusive, embracing the stranger and

39

giving refuge to the homeless? Will it be a caring America, nurturing the helpless and protecting the vulnerable?

"...The mark of a humane and progressive society is an ever more expansive definition of the community for which we accept responsibility... The pro-life movement is one with the movement for the emancipation of slaves. This is the continuation of the civil rights movement, for you are the champions of the most elementary civil, indeed human right – simply the right to be.

"There is another and authentically liberal vision of an America that is hospitable to the stranger, holding out arms of welcome to those who would share the freedom and opportunity we cherish. 'Give me your tired, your poor/Your huddled masses yearning to breathe free/The wretched refuse of your teeming shore/Send these, the homeless, tempest-tossed, to me/I lift my lamp beside the golden door.'

"The unborn child is the ultimate immigrant... The analogy between the unborn and the immigrant may seem strained. I fear, however, that it is painfully to the point."

According to Dr. And Mrs. J.C. Willke's 1988 *Handbook on Abortion*, a poll was conducted at the 1984 Democratic National Convention in San Francisco, CA, asking: "Should there be a Constitutional Amendment outlawing abortion?" It was found that only nine percent of all delegates to the Convention supported such an Amendment, even though it was supported by 46 percent of all Democrats nationwide.

The Reverend Jesse Jackson once observed that the "privacy" argument used in *Roe v. Wade* to justify abortion "was the premise of slavery. You could not protest the existence or treatment of slaves on the plantation because that was private and therefore outside of your right to be concerned." In an article appearing in the *Wall Street Journal* entitled "Are Black Leaders Listening to Black America?", J. Perkins wrote: "Black leaders react in traditional, knee-jerk liberal fashion to issues across the board, even though, in general, black Americans are decidedly conservative on a number of issues. The Black Caucus, for example, advocates a 'right' to abort, whereas 62% of blacks oppose abortion (National Opinion Research Center, 1984)."

According to Mary Meehan, "...abortion is a civil rights issue. Dick Gregory and many other blacks view abortion as a type of genocide." For every white baby killed by abortion, for example, two minority children die. Civil rights activist Fannie Lou Hamer (1917-1977) insisted, "The methods used to take human lives, such as abortion, the pill, the ring, etc., amount to genocide. I believe that legal abortion is legal murder."

According to Hamer, "These are still our children. And we still love these children. And after these babies are born we are not going to disband these children from their families, because these are other lives, they are... and I think these children have a right to live. And I think these mothers have a right to support them in a decent way."

A pamphlet distributed by Milwaukee SOUL (Save Our Unwanted Lives) points out that under current U.S. law, *corporations* are considered legal persons, while humans in prenatal development are denied this moral status.

In her essay, "Life and Peace," Juli Loesch wrote: "In a revealing article published in *Seven Days*, Michelle Magar suggests that the New Right's relationship with Right to Life has been 'more a marriage of convenience than true love.' She suggests that the anti-abortion position adds 'a certain moral luster' to the New Right, which otherwise has a distinctly different set of priorities (threatening war for the possession of Persian Gulf oil, and so forth). Magar points out that, in a practical sense, the New Right's concern for the unborn gives it access to the 'grassroots anti-abortion network of the Catholic Church – a ready-made constituency which they had so far never been able to win.'"

Public attitudes towards abortion were revealed in a March 1991 Gallup poll. 66 percent of those polled did not think financial hardships justify abortion. 68 percent did not think "abandonment by partner" is a valid reason to abort an unborn child.

The Center for Disease Control in Atlanta reported that over two-thirds of all women seeking abortions in 1983 were not using any kind of birth control, while 40 percent of all abortions that year were performed on women who had already had at least one before. Nonetheless, 88 percent of Americans polled said they opposed abortion as a "repeated means of birth control."

91 percent of Americans polled said they opposed abortion as a means of sex selection (prenatal sexual discrimination), while 69 percent supported parental

consent legislation and viability testing on fetuses after the fifth month of pregnancy. This is significant because only 58 percent of Americans are aware that *Roe v. Wade* legalized abortion during the entire nine months of pregnancy, and not just during the first trimester.

Informing a new mother about human prenatal development and the alternatives to abortion was supported by 86 percent of those polled, while 52 percent of the women polled felt the right to life of the unborn child outweighs the mother's freedom to kill.

The American public is only familiar with the conservative Republican opposition to abortion. Columnist Tom Goff called the 1992 Republican National Convention "a gathering of loonies." The intelligent, rational, secular, *liberal* opposition to abortion goes unreported by the popular news media.

Columnist Nat Hentoff of the *Village Voice*, a self-described "liberal Jewish atheist," wrote an article in 1988 entitled, "A Liberal's Journey to the Pro-Life Side." In a 1992 article entitled, "Pro-Life Feminists: Celebrating Life's Greatest Liberty," Hentoff wrote that R.W. Apple, Jr., in the *New York Times*, had described then governor of Pennsylvania Robert Casey as "a conservative Democrat."

According to Hentoff, however, Casey made Pennsylvania one of the first states to mandate help for young, disabled children (with $45 million for the first year). He set up a model child-care program for state workers; he had been pushing for family leave legislation; and he had put together a program to assure health care to every uninsured Pennsylvania child up to the age of six.

"This 'conservative' governor has been lauded by the National Women's Caucus for his persistence in naming women cabinet appointees (40 percent) and in increasing the participation of women and minorities in state construction contracts from one percent to 15 percent. He is also a friend of labor (a phrase that used to be said more often with regard to Democratic politicians).

"I asked Governor Casey how he felt being preserved in the *New York Times* Index as a conservative. Casey laughed. 'Well, that's the mind set of a good many people, in and out of the press. If you're pro-life, you must be conservative.'

"The press has been cautioned about its bent toward stereotyping pro-lifers," noted Hentoff. "...many readers and viewers have a decidedly limited sense of the diversity of pro-lifers. Feminists For Life of America, for example, includes women who came out of the civil rights and anti-war movements and now work for what they call 'a consistent ethic of life.'

"Rachel MacNair (president of Feminists For Life) has been arrested at least 17 times – for protesting against nuclear plants and nuclear weapons."

In a September 15, 1992 article appearing in the *Village Voice* entitled, "The Excommunication of Robert Casey," Hentoff observed that the Democratic Party had abandoned free speech by not allowing Casey to speak at the 1992 Democratic National Convention. According to Casey, "The Democratic National Committee has become a wholly owned subsidiary of the National Abortion Rights Action League."

Casey said he would strongly support Lynn Yeakel who was then running against Republican Senator Arlen Specter in Pennsylvania. Yeakel favors abortion but, Casey said, "we agree on all the other issues." Casey stated further that he would not leave the Democratic Party. The anti-abortion Republicans, he insisted, "drop the children at birth and do nothing for them after that."

Unlike Republicans, pro-life liberals advocate real social support for pregnant women and mothers. In *Pro-Life Feminism: Different Voices*, editor Gail Grenier Sweet calls for:

Easy access to contraception, sufficient maternity and paternity leaves, job protection, job-sharing and flex-time, aids to women who wish to stay home to raise young children, tax breaks and subsidies for women caring for elderly relatives at home, community based shelters for pregnant single women to learn parenting skills and finish their education, upgraded pension plans to alleviate the poverty faced by many elderly women, humane care of the handicapped and elderly in nursing homes, hospices for the terminally ill, medical care for infants born with handicaps, shelters for battered women, childcare programs, etc.

Similarly, in the December 1993 issue of *Harmony: Voices for a Just Future*, in an article entitled "How Will we Revere Life?", editor Rose Evans writes:

"This editor has long been aware of the relative success of the Dutch support system for pregnant women, compared to that of the U.S. The Dutch abortion rate is a minute fraction of the American. I believe the rate for young women in their teens is about one-twentieth of the U.S. rate. And this is done not so much by restrictive laws (although there are some restrictions) as by real social support for pregnant women and mothers.

"The situation for pregnant women in the U.S. who don't have assured income, family support and medical insurance is abysmal and getting worse. Choice is a joke. Women don't have money for decent food, decent housing, or decent medical care, nor adequate support after the child is born."

Some argue that abortion is a necessary evil to prevent the United States from becoming an overburdened "welfare state." At present, however, there are over two million couples and one million single people wishing to adopt. Figures from Planned Parenthood show welfare costs of $13,900 for each birth. Compare this to the figure of $50,000 each American ends up paying in taxes as an adult. Moreover, the average time a family stays on welfare is only 27 months.

Persons concerned about a return to "back-alley" abortions if abortion were made illegal again should first read *Aborting America* by Dr. Bernard Nathanson. 1983 data from the Bureau of Vital Statistics show one would have to go back to the pre-penicillin era to find more than 1,000 maternal deaths per year.

During 1965 to 1966, the period right before states began to legalize abortion, the number of total deaths were down to 120 per year. In 1970, the figure was 128 per year. A

Kinsey study in 1960 showed that 84 to 87 percent of all illegal abortions were performed by reputable physicians.

Dr. Mary Calderone of Planned Parenthood once stated, "Ninety percent of all illegal abortions are presently done by physicians."

The majority of pro-life activists also regard the mother seeking abortion as a *victim* and not a criminal. Looking back on over two hundred years of legal history, the American Center for Bioethics concluded that women have never been prosecuted for abortion; only the abortionists. This is analogous to our current laws which arrest drug dealers and prostitutes rather than their clientele. If we continue to imperfectly enforce laws like these against what are arguably victimless crimes, why can't we take steps towards protecting the human unborn?

One widespread argument against recognizing the humanity of the unborn, is that we must then oppose all forms of contraception, since this also means the destruction of human life. Sperm and egg, however, like saliva and other bodily excretions, are genetically identical to male and female respectively, while a newly formed human zygote is a separate individual human being, genetically distinct from both parents.

There is no environment anywhere in which an individual sperm or an egg cell could be placed and made to grow into an embryo, fetus, infant, toddler, adolescent, etc. Doing so would be as absurd as placing a nonfertile chicken egg into an incubator and expecting a chicken to hatch! Eating a *fertile* chicken egg, on the other hand, as all vegetarians know, effectively kills a chicken.

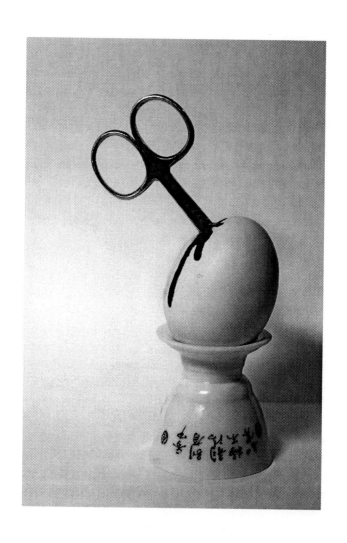

Similar reasoning prompted the federal government to enact a law imposing a $5,000 fine for destroying any fertilized bald eagle egg.

"Is birth control an abortion?"
"Definitely not. An abortion kills the life of a baby after it has begun."

---Planned Parenthood pamphlet
    August 1963

While there may be *religious* reasons to oppose contraception, divorce, fornication, homosexuality, masturbation, oral sex, etc. there are no rational, secular arguments against such practices.

Gays Against Abortion (now known as PLAGAL, or the Pro-Life Alliance of Gays and Lesbians) was formed in 1991. They issued a statement:

"We acknowledge that, from conception, the fetus is a human being entitled to basic rights, including the right to life. We hold that abortion denies that right and destroys that human being. We know first hand, from homophobia, what it is to have our rights denied... Like homophobia, abortion tries to get rid of the persons who are considered undesirable... We volunteer time and energy to pro-life pregnancy centers and pro-life agencies..."

Similarly, in the May 1992 issue of *Harmony: Voices for a Just Future*, in an article entitled, "Coming Out of the Closet for Life," Donna Marie Kearney wrote: "It is difficult to understand why so many gay and lesbian people can support the so-called 'woman's right' to abortion. While living as oppressed people, they are blind to the subversion of the rights of the unborn, the weakest and most powerless among us."

Kearney is a lesbian Christian peace activist, a member of the Faith and Resistance Community, and has been arrested in protest against nuclear weapons storage, and arrested along with Daniel Berrigan and others for trespassing at a Planned Parenthood building.

"Want to Stop Abortions?": asks the June 1995 newsletter for the Colorado Peace Mission in Boulder, CO. "Make them unnecessary. Provide *everyone* with: A choice of whether to have sex... and with whom; Comprehensive sex education; Non-coercive family planning; Safe, affordable birth control; Open, honest talk about sex; Loving parents..."

In a 1991 article entitled "When No News is Bias," Reverend James Burtchaell, a professor of theology at the University of Notre Dame, drew comparisons between civil disobedience directed against abortion clinics and "the far more controversial sit-ins and freedom marches of the 1960s, the raiding of draft board files in the 1970s, the denting of ICBM nose cones in the 1980s, the blockading of the South African Embassy in 1984..."

According to Reverend Burtchaell, these demonstrators had their rights violated: "A 72-year-old bishop in West Hartford, Connecticut, was seized, cuffed behind his back, then lifted from the ground by billy clubs between his wrists... 17 female college students had their clothes ripped off and were forced to walk in the nude, in some cases crawl.

"Some of them were sexually assaulted... arrested women were strip-searched and cavity searched; others were stripped to the waist and dragged through the jail by their bras with breasts exposed... prisoners in Atlanta were forbidden to pray together in jail...":

Reverend Burtchaell noted further that "whereas actor Martin Sheen was given three hours of community service for his 18th conviction for anti-nuclear protest, a first-time abortion protester in Fargo, North Dakota, was sent to prison for 21 months. Militant homosexuals who had invaded St. Patrick's Cathedral and disrupted Mass were fined $100; the organizers of the New York and other pro-life protests have been fined $450,000."

Anti-abortion clergy and protesters must be given the same level of respect (and equal time to air their views through the news media) given to animal rights activists, environmentalists, feminists, civil rights activists, anti-nuclear activists, anti-capital punishment activists, antiwar activists, "militant homosexuals," etc.

In These Times, a progressive political newspaper in Chicago observed in the late 1980s: "Our reaction to scenes of anti-abortion activists engaging in civil disobedience outside of clinics is similar to that of many on the Left: 'What are THEY doing using OUR tactics? One major factor may be uncomfortable for many of us to admit: that many of them ARE us.'"

The Seamless Garment Network (SGN) is a coalition of peace and justice organizations on the religious Left. The SGN takes a stand against war, abortion, poverty, racism, the arms race, the death penalty and euthanasia. Animal rights, like ecology, nuclear power, gun control, or the drug war, is a topic of serious discussion among SGN members. His Holiness the Dalai Lama has signed the SGN Mission Statement.

Carol Crossed, then Executive Director of the SGN, wrote in 1994:

"In the last 27 years, I have engaged in civil disobedience and risked arrest in over 20 demonstrations around issues as varied as civil rights in Washington, DC; anti-Vietnam War actions; and sleeping outside the City Hall in Rochester, NY to call attention to the plight of the homeless. Most recently, I was arrested in opposition to the Gulf War. Five of these arrests were in opposition to aborting children. Rescues are not a monolithic expression by a single group. Many participants, even leaders, are feminists, Quakers, and Pacifists from Catholic Worker communities."

On January 21, 1994, the U.S. Supreme Court ruled unanimously that the sanctions of the Racketeer Influenced and Corrupt Organizations Act (RICO) could be applied to anti-abortion protesters. According to Carol Crossed, "It is an inescapable fact that activists today engage in acts of civil disobedience remarkably similar to some of the acts of pro-life protesters which NOW (the National Organization for Women) would like to transform into federal felons...

"Environmentalists chain themselves to trees; plowshares activists damage warheads; and animal rights activists sit in at stockyard feed lots. A current bill (HR 1815) called 'Hunter Harassment' is under consideration which would not only criminalize actions against hunters – assaults, seizing guns, blocking entrances to hunting grounds, etc. – but speech directed at hunters as well.

"A *Washington Post* editorial 'Shouting and Shooting' (12/3/93) says, 'The point of picketing, protests, demonstrations and boycotts is to make people who are targets so uncomfortable that they will change their politics or behavior. So it is with the opponents of hunting, as it has been with civil rights, labor unions and abortion protesters.'"

When the RICO decision was issued, Carol Crossed saw it as a threat to the whole range of nonviolent protest, and warned others of the threat that the RICO decision posed to all forms of nonviolent protest and peaceful dissent.

Signers of a newspaper ad protesting the decision included Erwin Knoll, editor of *The Progressive*; Daniel Berrigan, S.J.; Philip Berrigan; Liz McAlister; Leonard Peltier, American Indian Movement; Joseph Lowery, President of the Southern Christian Leadership Conference; civil rights leader Will Campbell; environmentalist Wendell Berry and others.

Organizations signing included the International Black Women's Network; the Fund for Animals; Koininea Partners; People for the Ethical Treatment of Animals (PETA); *Sojourners* and others.

Anti-nuclear plowshares activists have met with Operation Rescue activists and even "pro-life" and "pro-choice" activists have met to find common ground. Why shouldn't there be an ongoing discussion between animal rights and anti-abortion activists?

Columnist Colman McCarthy, a liberal Catholic writer, is an example of an animal rights advocate who may literally be called "pro-life." McCarthy teaches filled-to-capacity classes on nonviolence in high schools and colleges in the Washington, DC area. He speaks eloquently about the rights of "our fellow Earthians, whom we call animals.

"How many of you had a corpse for lunch today?" he asks his students. "What part of an animal did you eat? A leg? A rib? I never call it meat – that's just a euphemism. You know why I avoid dairy products and eggs? Because they're sexist; it's the females in the barns and henhouses. What do you think of that?"

McCarthy has even drawn fire for advocating vegetarianism. Senator Jesse Helms (R-NC) once accused McCarthy of having communist ties, after he had urged Americans to skip turkey and eat bulgur at Thanksgiving. In one of his columns, he wrote that American society "chews on the cadavers" of nine million animals a day, and quoted Nobel Prize winning author Isaac Bashevis Singer on the subject of vegetarianism.

McCarthy writes about public education, the violence of our meat-producing and chemical-agriculture industries, and the wasted millions of dollars spent on the military buildup and high school ROTC programs. He has also expressed opposition to abortion.

"Have you heard the new pro-choice strategy?" he asked in the spring of 1989 after a huge abortion rally in Washington, DC. "Now they're all saying nobody *wants* abortion, but that it's important to keep the option open." (He shakes his head) "That's like a general who says he doesn't like war, but wants to keep it as an option, just in case. You don't find peace through war, and you don't enhance life through killing babies."

Labor leader Cesar Chavez of the United Farm Workers, like Colman McCarthy, was also an ethical vegetarian opposed to abortion.

Loss of Life Compared

Each ribbon signifies 50,000 American deaths. War statistics are as reported by CNN, cited from the Department of Defense and the Department of Veterans Affairs. Abortion statistics provided by the Alan Guttmacher Institute, Planned Parenthood's research organization.

Civil War 1861-1865   **498,332 Deaths**

Ꝝ Ꝝ Ꝝ Ꝝ Ꝝ Ꝝ Ꝝ Ꝝ Ꝝ

World War I 1917-1918   **116,516 Deaths**

Ꝝ Ꝝ

World War II 1941-1945   **405,399 Deaths**

Ꝝ Ꝝ Ꝝ Ꝝ Ꝝ Ꝝ Ꝝ Ꝝ

Vietnam War 1964-1975   **58,200 Deaths**

Ꝝ

Persian Gulf War 1990-1991   **382 Deaths**

< Ꝝ

War on Terror 10/7/2001-12/12/2005 **2397 Deaths**
(Includes Afghanistan, Iraq, and other theaters)

< Ꝝ

Abortion 1973-2002   **42 million Deaths**

ƒ x 840, or:

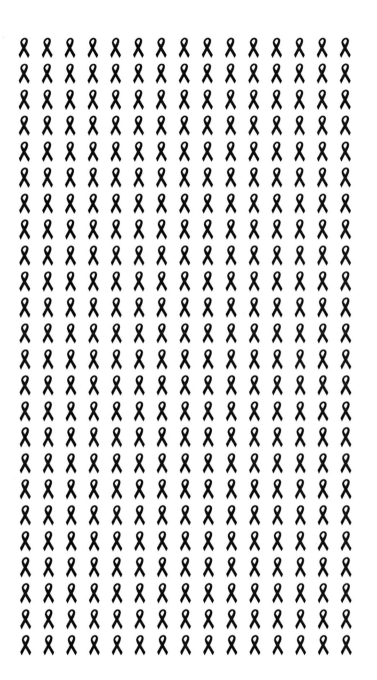

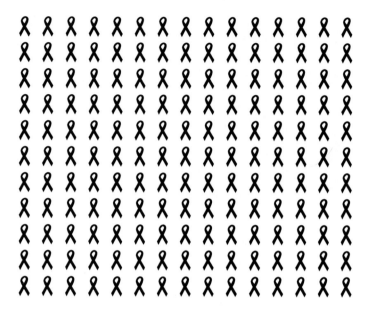

According to the Alan Guttmacher Institute's March 18 2005 report, there were 1.29 million abortions in 2002 – a decrease from an estimated 1.36 million in 1996. Using the lower of the two figures, we would add 25 ribbons for each year:

The death toll caused by war is indeed tragic, but the death toll caused by abortion is much greater. Only humanity's holocaust of the animal kingdom (45 billion annually) results in a far greater loss of life.

Vegetarianism: It's Pro-Life

"The reasons for legal intervention in favor of children apply not less strongly to the case of those unfortunate slaves – the animals."

---John Stuart Mill

Henry Bergh, founder of the American Society for the Prevention of Cruelty to Animals (ASPCA), successfully prosecuted a woman for child abuse in 1873, at a time when children had no legal protection, under the then currently existing animal protection statutes. This case started the child-saving crusade around the world.

A rational case exists for the rights of preborn humans. The case for animal rights is equally compelling. Animals are highly complex creatures, possessing a brain, a central nervous system and a sophisticated mental life.

Animals actually *suffer* at the hands of their human tormentors and exhibit such "human" behaviors and feelings as fear and physical pain, defense of their children, pair bonding, group/tribal loyalty, grief at the loss of loved ones, joy, jealousy, competition, territoriality, and cooperation.

Dr. Tom Regan, the foremost intellectual leader of the animal rights movement and author of *The Case for Animal Rights*, notes that animals "have beliefs and desires; perception, memory, and a sense of the future, including their own future; and emotional life together with feelings of pleasure and pain; preference and welfare interests; the ability to initiate action in pursuit of their desires and goals; a psychophysical identity over time; and an individual welfare in the sense that their experiential life fares well or ill for them, logically independent of their utility for others and logically independent of their being the object of anyone else's interests."

While it is known that the feminist movement originally opposed abortion as "child-murder" (Susan B. Anthony's words) and as a form of violence that women are forced to turn to in a patriarchal society, a society that shows virtually no concern or respect for new mothers, it is generally not known that many of the early American feminists – including Lucy Stone, Amelia Bloomer, Susan B. Anthony and Elizabeth Cady Stanton – were connected with the 19th century animal welfare movement. Together, they would meet with anti-slavery editor Horace Greeley to toast "Women's Rights and Vegetarianism."

Many of the early American feminists thus saw animal rights as the logical next step in social progress after women's rights and civil rights. Count Leo Tolstoy similarly described ethical vegetarianism as social progress:

"And there are ideas of the future, of which some are already approaching realization and are obliging people to change their way of life and to struggle against the former ways: such ideas in our world as those of freeing the laborers, of giving equality to women, of ceasing to use flesh-food, and so on."

The case for animal rights and vegetarianism should be readily understandable to the millions of Americans opposed to abortion on demand. "Although I may disagree with some of its underlying principles," writes pro-life activist Karen Swallow Prior, "there is much for me, an anti-abortion activist, to respect in the animal rights movement. Animal rights activists, like me, have risked personal safety and reputation for the sake of other living beings. Animal rights activists, like me, are viewed by many in the mainstream as fanatical wackos, ironically exhorted by irritated passerby to 'Get a Life!'

"Animal rights activists, like me, place a higher value on life than on personal comfort and convenience, and in balancing the sometimes competing interests of rights and responsibilities, choose to err on the side of compassion and nonviolence."

Both the anti-abortion and animal rights movements consider their cause a form of social progress, like the abolition of human slavery or the emancipation of women. Leaders in both movements have even compared themselves to the abolitionists who sought to end human slavery.

Dr. J.C. Willke, former head of National Right to Life, entitled a book *Abortion and Slavery*. Like abortion opponents drawing a parallel between the *Dred Scott* decision and *Roe v. Wade*, Dr. Tom Regan also draws a parallel between human and animal slavery in *The Case for Animal Rights*:

"The very notion that farm animals should continue to be viewed as legal property must be challenged. To view them in this way implies that we cannot make sense of viewing them as legal persons. But the history of the law shows only too well, and too painfully, how arbitrary the law can be on this crucial matter. Those humans who were slaves were not recognized as legal persons in pre-Civil War America.

"There is no reason to assume that because animals are not presently accorded this status that they cannot intelligibly be viewed in this way or that they should not be. If our predecessors had made this same assumption in the case of human slaves, the legal status of these human beings would have remained unchanged."

Both movements see themselves extending human rights to a disenfranchised class of beings. Both movements claim to be speaking on behalf of a class of beings unable to defend themselves from oppression. Both movements compare the mass destruction of, in one case the human unborn, and in the other case, the mass killing of animals, to the Nazi Holocaust.

Both movements have components that engage in nonviolent civil disobedience and both have their militant factions: Operation Rescue and the Animal Liberation Front. Both have picketed the homes of physicians who either experiment upon animals or perform abortions. The controversial use of human fetal tissue and embryonic stem cells for medical research brings these two causes even closer together.

Both movements are usually depicted in the popular news media as extremists, fanatics, terrorists, etc. who violate the law. But both movements also have their intelligentsia: moral philosophers, physicians, clergymen, legal counsel, etc.

Feminist writer Carol J. Adams notes the parallels between the two movements: "A woman attempts to enter a building. Others, massed outside, try to thwart her attempt. They shout at her, physically block her way, frantically call her names, pleading with her to respect life. Is she buying a fur coat or getting an abortion?"

The Fur Information Council of America asks: "If fashion isn't about freedom of choice, what is? Personal choice is not just a fur industry issue. It's everybody's issue." Like the abortion debate, lines are drawn. "Freedom of choice" vs. taking an innocent life. "Personal lifestyle" vs. violating another's rights.

Animal rights activists have even proven themselves to be "anti-choice" depending upon the issue. A letter in *The Animals' Voice Magazine*, for example, states: "Exit polls in Aspen, Colorado, after the failed 1989 fur ban was voted on, found that most people were against fur but wanted people to have a choice to wear it. Instead of giving in, we should take the offensive and state in no uncertain terms that to abuse and kill animals is wrong, period! There is no choice because another being had to suffer to produce that item... an eventual ban on fur would be impossible if we tell people that they have some sort of 'choice' to kill... remember, no one has the right to choose death over life for another being."

Similarly, a letter in *Veg-News* reads: "I did have some concerns about [the] Veg Psych column which asserted that we must respect a non-vegan's 'right to choose' her/his food. While I would never advocate intolerance (quite the opposite actually), arguing that we have a 'right to choose' when it comes to eating meat, eggs, and dairy is akin to saying we have a 'right to choose' to beat dogs, harass wildlife, and torture cats. Each is a clear example of animal cruelty, whether we're the perpetrators ourselves, or the ones who pay others to commit the violence on our behalf. Clearly, we have the ability to choose to cause animal abuse, but that doesn't translate into a right to make that choice."

Recognizing the rights of another class of beings, of course, limits our freedoms and our choices, and requires a change in our personal lifestyle. The abolition of (human) slavery is good example of this. Both movements, however, appear to be imposing their own personal moral convictions upon the rest of our secular society.

Animal rights activists point out the health hazards associated with meat, eggs, and dairy products, while anti-abortion activists try to educate the public about the link between abortion and breast cancer. The threat of "overpopulation" is frequently used to justify abortion as birth control. On a vegetarian diet, however, the world could easily support a population several times its present size. The world's cattle alone consume enough to feed 8.7 billion humans.

Both movements make use of similar political tactics, such as economic boycotting. Both movements make use of graphic photos or videos of abortion victims or tortured animals. Both movements speak of respecting life and of compassion. Both movements cite studies that unnecessary violence towards an oppressed class of beings leads to worse forms of violence in human society – this is known as the "slippery slope." The term was coined by Malcolm Muggeridge, a pro-life vegetarian.

Anti-abortion activists, for example, consider abortion the ultimate form of child abuse, and claim that since abortion was legalized, child abuse rates have risen dramatically. Acceptance of abortion, they argue, leads to a devaluation of human life, and paves the way towards acceptance of infanticide and euthanasia. Animal rights activists, likewise, compare the lives of animals to those of young human children, and insist that a lack of respect for the rights of animals brutalizes humans into insensitivity towards one another.

In his Pulitzer Prize nominated book, *Diet for a New America*, for example, author John Robbins writes of a Soviet study, published in *Ogonyok*, which found that over 87 percent of a group of violent criminals had, as children, burned, hanged or stabbed domestic animals. An American study by Dr. Stephen Kellert of Yale found that children who abuse animals have a much higher likelihood of becoming violent criminals. A 1997 study by the Massachusetts Society for the Prevention of Cruelty to Animals (MSPCA) reported that children convicted of animal abuse are five times more likely to commit violence against other humans than are their peers, and four times more likely to be involved in acts against property.

Pro-lifers have reason to be especially concerned about violence towards animals. Animals are sentient beings possessing many mental capacities comparable to those of young human children. If we fail to see them as part of our moral community, how will we ever embrace humans in their most primitive stages of development? Anti-abortionists look in horror as an entire class of humans are systematically stripped of their rights, executed, and even used as tools for medical research. Yet this is what we humans have been doing to animals for millennia.

Marjorie Spiegel, author of *The Dreaded Comparison: Human and Animal Slavery*, writes: "All oppression and violence is intimately and ultimately linked, and to think that we can end prejudice and violence to one group without ending prejudice and violence to another is utter folly."

Mostly religious in nature, the anti-abortion movement will need to become completely secular, as it attempts to convince the courts, the legislatures, philosophers, ethicists and universities that human zygotes and embryos should be regarded as legal persons. Conversely, the animal rights movement is secular and nonsectarian, but – like the civil rights movement – will need the inspiration, blessings and support of organized religion to help end injustices towards animals. The Reverend Marc Wessels, Executive Director of the International Network for Religion and Animals (INRA), made this observation on Earth Day, 1990:

"It is a fact that no significant social reform has yet taken place in this country without the voice of the religious community being heard. The endeavors of the abolition of slavery; the women's suffrage movement; the emergence of the pacifist tradition during World War I; the struggle to support civil rights, labor unions and migrant farm workers;

and the anti-nuclear and peace movements have all succeeded in part because of the power and support of organized religion. Such authority and energy is required by individual Christians and the institutional church today if the liberation of animals is to become a reality."

At a speech before the National Right to Life Convention in Cherry Hill, New Jersey, on July 15, 1982, Reverend Richard John Neuhaus of the Evangelical Lutheran Church said:

"...The mark of a humane and progressive society is an ever more expansive definition of the community for which we accept responsibility... The pro-life movement is one with the movement for the emancipation of slaves. This is the continuation of the civil rights movement, for you are the champions of the most elementary civil, indeed human right – simply the right to be."

While there are indeed similarities between the present day anti-abortion movement and the anti-slavery movement of centuries past, the pro-life movement, actually, also has a lot in common with the animal protection movement – a fact which pro-lifers should readily acknowledge. The animal rights movement should be supported by all caring Americans.

Ingrid Newkirk, Executive Director of People for the Ethical Treatment of Animals, admitted in an interview with Dennis Prager, that the animal rights movement is divided on the issue of abortion. Where should an animal rights activist stand with regards to abortion? Mohandas Gandhi, India's great apostle of nonviolence, once wrote, "It seems to me clear as daylight that abortion would be a crime." C.S. Lewis and other Christians have acknowledged that denying rights to animals merely because they do not exhibit the same level of rational thought most humans exhibit upon reaching full development means denying rights to the mentally handicapped, the senile, and many other classes of humans as well. Herein lies the basis for better understanding and cooperation between two movements seeking liberty and justice for all.

Conclusion

"I am struck by how knee-jerk the liberal/progressive community is on the necessity of legal abortions," writes Timothy Shipe of Westerville, Ohio, in the June 2003 issue of *The Progressive*. "On every other issue, the progressive community looks at the parties involved, assesses the humanity, the vulnerability, the justice, the balance of power, and then weighs in on the side of the underdog. Every issue, that is, except for abortion.

"The day I accept as 'progressive' the anti-human practice of willful abortion is the day I say OK to unjust war, unfettered capitalist exploitation of people and the environment, capital punishment, ethnic cleansing, and so forth."

Opposition to abortion can be found across the political spectrum. A national poll by Wirthlin Worldwide on the evening of the 1998 elections found that 38 percent of all Democrats (and 40 percent of Democrat women) oppose abortion. A national poll released by the Center for Gender Equality (a women's think tank headed by former Planned Parenthood executive director Faye Wattleton), in January 1999, found that a majority of American women do not support legalized abortion on demand. 53 percent of female respondents to the poll said abortion should be allowed only in cases of rape, incest, to save a mother's life or not at all, up from 45 percent in 1996.

A Zogby International poll in August 1999 found that the majority of Americans recognize that abortion destroys a new individual human life (52 percent versus 36 percent), oppose partial-birth abortions (56.4 percent versus 32 percent), are opposed to tax-funded partial-birth abortions (71 percent to 23 percent), and think parents should be notified if their minor child seeks an abortion (78 percent).

The abortion controversy is analogous to the Vietnam War. By the late 1960s, both the right and the left came to agree that the war was wrong; they merely advocated different strategies for ending it. The real losers on this issue are the 1.5 million annual victims of prenatal homicide, and the spineless politicians afraid to speak out against the madness.

On secular, human rights grounds, the American Left should take a stand against abortion.

About the Author

  Writer and activist Vasu Murti was born and raised in
Southern California in a family of South Indian Brahmins.
He holds degrees in Physics and Applied Mathematics from
the University of California. He has written articles on a
number of different topics, including secularism, science
versus religion, animal rights, nuclear power, handgun
control, Buddhism, abortion, illegal immigration, and drug
legalization. He is a regular contributor to *Harmony:
Voices for a Just Future*, a "consistent ethic" publication on
the religious left. Vasu is a "card-carrying" member of the
ACLU, Feminists For Life, Amnesty International, and
People for the Ethical Treatment of Animals.

Printed in the United States
84710LV00001B/181/A

9 780977 223435